King Street Blues

Denis Fitzpatrick

Thanks to:
Agent Violet

First Published by:
Independence Jones
guerrilla press division
Po Box 207 Petersham 2049
NSW, Australia

Publishers note:
All care has been taken to protect the identities of people connected with this re-telling.

Contents

Chapter One

~

Naturally Emerging From

Living on the streets was wonderful, with, of course, its fair share of woe.

In essence, I went into my previous five years life of homelessness (1994-1999) with my eyes open, hoping to be finally confronted with great depths within myself, naturally emerging from an environment devoid of stimuli. I have discovered these tremendous depths, as outlined in most of my previous short stories and anthologies and am still surprised that they were discovered through a life of wilful depravity.

Anyway.

When I was almost twenty-two I decided to go to Melbourne, a city that I had visited with my family when younger. The city accordingly impressed itself into my perspective as a result and that bright autumn morning being so beautiful I decided to go back there and fulfil the first of my goals and set up base in this artists' city.

'Stan, I'm going to Melbourne now. Do you want to come?' I was at my first share-house, in Redfern and had just barged in on my old friend.

I have known Stanley Nilsson for eleven years now and despite his anarchism, he has always been unable to understand my somewhat eccentric manners. This bothers me greatly.

Nevertheless he remains generous and offered me a room in his share house at a discount price, considering that I was a brother of one of his high school friends and the fact that I was taking flight from the nest.

He was still asleep on that mild, autumn morning in 1994 and after I repeated my suggestion, he found it ridiculous. It's only now that I can see that he would find this so.

The train station was very close by and after changing at Central and waiting until about 1:30 pm, I was on my way to the heart of the Garden State.

Until the ticket inspector introduced herself to me on approach to Campbelltown.

'Can I see your ticket please, sir.'

'I've accidentally left it behind.'

'That's okay; what's your surname and I'll just check you off.'

Ah, I see. That a problem which I would have to be very, very lucky to fix.

'Actually, I haven't got a ticket,' I began in a reasonable enough tone. 'Can I pay for it in Melbourne?' That was another problem, but no matter, no matter.

'I'm sorry sir,' although she didn't look sorry, 'only paying passengers beyond this point.'

'But I can pay at my destination! Surely, we can sort something out here?'

'Sorry sir, company policy: booked passengers only may pass the Inspector.'

Whom let me off at Campbelltown.

And being thus abandoned of transport towards my focused fancy, without money and only a loaf of nut-bread for sustenance in my sports bag, I decided that reaching Melbourne must be reasonably expected of a developed nation's citizen, if that's what he/she wished. The thing to do now was find a way towards this expected success.

So I experimented with hitchhiking. I prefer the index finder method, rather than the traditional thumb, which I think just looks more interesting. What works even better is when one employs some dancing, exotic rhythm in that ancient seeking gesture. This causes lots of people to honk as they pass by and a high percentage of Ferals will stop to help you out.

The ultimate effect of all this shimmying and alternative lifestyles is that one truly physically feels on the road of some great adventure, mingling with others in the midst of secret ceremonies.

But now that I think about it, psychos are also usually somewhat more charismatic and 'unique', preferring the exotic.

My first lift was heading the wrong way but he let me off at the Hume Highway and pointed out which direction was south.

Thus, and fully cognisant of such, I was all alone in the middle of nowhere, heading vaguely south. After trying the thumb, I reverted to the jigging digit approach and walked along with my head bent in order to avoid the feeling that the sky was falling.

I really wanted to get to Melbourne, and I'm used to getting what I want.

After about an hour or three-quarters a sedan pulled up in front of me.

'G'day,' I said through the passenger window to the scraggy male driver.

'G'day. Where are you off to?'

'Melbourne.'

'I can give you a lift to a petrol station where there are truckies headed there.'

'Cool.' So I hopped in, wondering why people are generally frightened of hitchhiking. It's no riskier than most other activities.

Soon enough, with a makeshift sign gleaned from the service station, I was picked up by a middle-aged American couple, out here on holidays. And wouldn't you know it they were heading exactly in my direction.

'Yeah, well we saw your sign,' happily recounted the tanned matriarch. 'And Robert said, "wouldn't it be fun if we picked him up."'

The husband duly concurred and added,

'I'll try anything once.'

I can't truly recall their names presently and now that I think of it, I remember them actually being a sister and a brother. The sister had a tub of cornflake cookies in the open glove box which were among the tastiest things that I've ever eaten. She would have let me eat them all, which she even suggested but my manners aren't that eccentric.

The conversation along the way was relatively low key and I couldn't escape the feeling that I had to sell myself to them to appear intelligent, witty and worldly.

Falling asleep for most of the journey impressed me with no-one. I feel especially sad for this as we stopped off along the way, here and there, for a beer, or something to eat. They paid for everything and yet I still fell asleep on them without even wanting to relate to them on any fundamental, meaningful par.

'Melbourne!' announced our bright, cheery female host. It was early evening, dark and drizzling. They dropped me off as soon as possible, or so I felt and having located the direction of the University of Melbourne, decided to sleep there for the night in some warm nook of a building.

I shivered all night, trying not to think of how I was going to survive in a strange city, with no resources except for my welfare payments which I wasn't presently entitled to anyway considering that I had moved to a state of higher unemployment.

I was greeted the following morn by a female security guard who radioed her supervisor that she 'could have discovered a body.' In a sense, it was just that: only a body, with only the barest of clothing, grasping at shadows.

But she was thankfully disavowed of her hypothesis when I bolted upright and let the thin blanket slowly drop from my head and torso. Slowly I turned to face her.

'Boo!'

She looked duly frightened and began backing away from me.

I had a quiet laugh and then informed her horrified mien.

'It's okay sister, I'm not dead. Just cold.'

'Are you sure?'

'Well, I wouldn't know if I was dead but I would know if I was cold.'

She looked at me quizzically.

'Are you a student here?'

'No, just a traveller. I slept here last night.'

'You'll have to continue on your way then. The University can't help you.'

'Not a problem.'

She left then, in her security car and I packed my useless blanket away.

I prepared breakfast and realised that I was technically homeless, with absolutely nowhere to claim as niche, no money to get such for over a week and nothing substantial to eat now, or in the near future.

I finished my meagre breakfast and talked myself away from the relative safety of the campus to solve my present predicament.

'Ask and you shall receive.'

Chapter Two

~

The Basic Problem

The basic problem here is money. With a reasonable amount I can afford rent and food. I'll pay the bond in a few weeks.

So the destination chose itself: the DSS, the Department of Social Security, now known as centrelink. I was already registered with them but I had to explain why I had moved to a state of presently higher unemployment in order to remain eligible for payments. The office was in North Melbourne and I stumbled my way there on a few free tram rides. I simply told the conductor that I had just got here from Sydney, without any money and could he please tell me how to get to the nearest DSS? This was a tactic I sometimes reverted to in fey moods during the Melbourne almost constant cold and drizzle. And don't forget the chill factor.

When I finally arrived I encountered a room full of people and a long queue.

I hope the rest of the world hasn't gone crazy as well?

I noticed the ticket machine, took a ticket and then a seat.

I was called up at about 2 pm After taking my name and client number he quickly asked the obvious.

'Why have you moved to somewhere worse off?'

'The market that I am looking for work in is bigger here in Melbourne.'

He looked at me sceptically.

'And what industry is that?'

'I'm a writer.'

'Have you published anything?' The classical response.

'Not yet.'

He looked back at his monitor, adjusting his glasses and clicked away to the tune of an unknown pattern.

'Well, Mr. Fitzpatrick, it would appear from your records that you indeed have literary intention and I personally agree that Melbourne has more potential for the truly creative than Sydney. In light of which, we can re-register you and arrange a pre-payment against your next payment, if you wish?'

I was flabbergasted.

'Yes, certainly, that would be perfect.'

And after a few short hours of unbelieving impatience, I still doubted the printout of my balance: $140.00.

Thank you, Australia. You made my dream come true.

*

But being on the verge of a home didn't protect me from the constant drizzle of raindrops. And I was always out in that rain, looking in pubs, share-houses, on lampposts, anywhere, for some wholesome roof somewhere.

To no avail. For some reason, no-one would have me. A possible explanation as to why, in hindsight, was that I had not really considered the need to bathe. If there were any available facilities for such. Anyway the rain was currently taking care of that.

As to clothes, that was a luxury if you don't know what an op shop is.

I tried for two weeks to get a room somewhere and eventually decided to remain staying at a Hostel that was advertised at the DSS office in North Melbourne: Ozanam House, $5 a night. They let me stay there on credit and to this day have not asked me at all for repayment for about three or four months of residency.

Food was included free and almost constantly and I personally thought that it was reasonable quality. Breakfast time was the best, with fruit, milk, cereal, one glass of orange juice and always a meat dish of some sort. This last got me out of bed every morning, late, but in time to partake of their offering. It also gave me the energy to get out into the city to try and write some new short stories in the State Library of Victoria.

This last choice of 'office' naturally reflected my grand ambitions which were to come true. These wishes came true when I began to self-publish, in 2002, about seven years ago now. Towards the end of my first summer I had started selling some of my individual stories and anthologies to passers-by. Two of my customers, who worked behind the counter in a home wares shop in Newtown, returned for a new story that I was selling and the female of the pair, I vividly remember her saying (after she introduced herself and the shop she worked in) that,

'We both think that you're one of the great authors.'

Famous! At last!

Not only that but in about the warmth of 2003–2004, while selling my books at a jury-rigged stall on King Street, Newtown, several customers approached to purchase a book because of an article that they had read about my business in *The Sydney Morning Herald*. It was a very positive article and from some customers' responses it was a glowing report about my endeavours.

I later had a regular customer, Darren, confirm that he too had read the article and that it was indeed an enthusiastic commendation of my unique marketing style, as well as the stories' literary merits.

I had made it.

But that did take a while.

Anyway.

When Ozanam House unreproachfully pointed out to me about six weeks later that they could not reasonably be expected to carry me any further, completely gratis, I saw their point. Through them I soon found a room in Moonee Ponds for only $50.00 a week. In Sydney, the same would be about $80.00 in 1994 dollars.

I remained at this new address for about two weeks and only came out at night.

To write.

Under soft light.

Creating.

Unfortunately though, my food (Weet-Bix) ran out one night (my coffee had long been gone) and one of the neighbour's rooms caught fire the next night.

I saw this as a sign.

I left, and returned to Ozanam.

Feeling guilty though for living rent-free but with nowhere else to turn to of my own, I decided to reclaim the streets, while attempting to discover there Reasonable Definition.

Or so my reason expected.

Thus, exactly two freezing weeks before my 22nd birthday, I told my social worker, Julie, at Ozanam, that I was going to live on the streets.

Julie had a stress dummy on her desk, prominently displayed, which she claimed to never need, keeping it there more as a talking point. Her desk was neat and tidy with one of those 'You don't have to be crazy to work here...' signs. It was funny at the time.

'Why do you want to be homeless?' she asked, after making two coffees.

I could not answer. My reasons were subconsciously clear but I had not admitted to them yet. I answered.

'I think I'm on a quest.'

Of course this sudden belief in one's great importance is also a sign of schizophrenia. Yet Julie simply smiled at my response, somewhat sadly and ironically, having become familiar with my philosophical turn of mind.

'I can't stop you from doing what you want but I suggest you see our psychologist before you leave.'

'I'd rather not.'

We finished our coffee and Julie eventually bid me adieu. I already had my bag packed, with the same blanket that I arrived with and so headed directly out of the complex deliberately sure not to look behind me.

Where to next, with nowhere to go?

Chapter Three

~

Being Called Back

I was beginning to agree with the chilly winds and droplets that I was crazy. There is nothing romantic about shivering in a strange city constantly being exposed to the elements.

I realised this soon enough.

Thus, for the rest of my eight week stay in Melbourne, I slept in back alleys (often having to oust a resident litter of alley cats), driveways, building sites, parks and wherever else that looked safe for the night. I always avoided sleeping under cars and trucks despite the overnight shelter that they provided because Stan had already discussed this danger, saying that there are some homeless people who die every year from being accidentally run over from unexpectedly travelling motor vehicles. Even sleeping near them is dangerous, as one can so easily roll into hazard's way.

Building sites are also dangerous but the workers usually kicked me out at 5 am

There is also a suburban myth, which I was told by another friend, that a full edition of *The Age*, or similar, is quite a good blanket when one is open to the elements and when spread out accordingly. This is definitely not true, despite how many copies you use. The eventual result is that one winds up with a thorough litter of very good journalism, another guarded, sleepless, goose bumped night and a guilty conscious at wanting to leave the mess behind as some sort of revenge upon society.

Having enough to eat was not a problem, especially living so close to the free feed at Ozanam. I had my DSS Newstart Allowance and lunch and dinner was just a question of timing. I was still not willing to try the share-house or pub scene again though, not after having already received constant, consistent, promise-laden rejections – it's hard enough having good publishers rejecting me, let alone these suspiciously friendly strangers.

The sustenance that I tended to survive on (choosing to eat sparingly of the free food available) largely consisted of pasties, hot dogs, chocolates, yogurt and juices. Naturally enough, sitting outside a 7-Eleven one cold, bright night, I noticed that I was putting on weight. My top jeans button had just popped. It must have been under stress for several days for it to have popped so violently, with the sound of a miniature Big Bang.

This problem soon solved itself with the abstinence from that Great Aussie Pie and assorted pastries. And the chocolates. And with a sensible diet of sandwiches, rolls, the odd burger and regular exercise, I felt naturally more energetic, positive, still seeing my isolation as special.

Of course I could have afforded a backpackers hostel but I was simply too young, just turned 22 and too immature to even know that they existed.

Anyway.

After several sleepless weeks where all of my senses were scanning for trouble I discovered the ability to sleep in the bright, warm sun of an unexpected heat wave that was now over the city, and to get around in the night without being lonely.

The main trick there was to go into the city centre and find an all-night pub. Get yourself a beer and look for someone interesting to talk to.

I did this though only some of the time, preferring mostly to quietly absorb the warmth and mild glow of the atmosphere.

When the heat wave ended though it caught me by surprise as I had not naturally countered the inevitable removal of my cosy spot in some centrally located park, whose name I can't recall any more (I once woke up there to find someone had left me a set of sandwiches during my sleep).

Homelessness was not a path. I was prepared to go back to Sydney now, rather than face a well fed future of living in the rain.

It was the sleeping in the rain that eventually decided me.

*

Stan was not in Sydney, having left a couple of days before my arrival, for holidays in Melbourne.

I couldn't expect my parents to put me up, not after my very dramatic flight from the nest and Stan was the only one of my friends with enough contacts to get me a room somewhere on a short term basis, cheaply and instantly.

I probably should have let him know that I was returning but we all learn something every day, don't we?

I spent the intervening time at another hostel for the homeless, but like I said earlier, I'm not used to having to wait for what I want and so could not spend the time waiting productively. I wrote a bit but it was mainly poetry, short and containing everything that I felt needed to be said. I left a few copies behind and they were duly picked up.

*

Two weeks later my housing was sorted, as expected but there was another problem becoming very prominent to me.

Essentially, I was beginning to hear voices in my head and became utterly convinced that this was a sign of my immense magickal potential. I can't remember now exactly what these young male and female voices were saying. I have a recollection of them being very conversational – pointing things out, reminding me of how much money that I had left, even suggesting clothes to wear that I would see advertised in a window.

I drifted between a few more share-houses but no-one – except Stan and his girlfriend at the time, Treyna, knew that I was hearing voices and beginning to explore the possibility of my psychic ability.

I could explain it to no-one though, despite how much I saw that I needed to reveal this phenomenon so I spent all of my time locked in my various rooms, listening and talking with the voices whom all said nothing about my goal to be psychic.

These voices, coupled with a blue receipt of mine from the hostel that I had stayed upon my return to Sydney, led me back to the streets. The receipt had blown from Kings Cross and found me exactly six months later in Chippendale.

Clearly this was a sign calling me back to my mission, to maybe as the voices put it:

'SAVE THE UNIVERSE'S BACON!'

I still can't rationally explain how it found me. I can clearly remember throwing it away soon after receiving it at the hostel.

I also knew that this apparent 'sign from God' was also another self-fulfilling prophecy.

Thus I faced the decision, after being called back to my quest – do I go willingly, or with a struggle?

I returned home, packed my bags and left a note for Stan,

'GOING HOMELESS AGAIN!'

I didn't take a loaf of bread from the kitchen this time believing that I had been demanding enough with the last one for Melbourne.

I left and caught a train back to Kings Cross. To find some way of truly verifying Life, since it has always been cancelled by Death.

Chapter Four

~

By Liberty Discovered

The Domain, in Sydney, is a great place to camp out in. There are plenty of large, bushy trees, if the bunk-bed is your style. For the more traditional there are a few rocky nooks which provide a perfect windbreak and reasonable privacy from the plethora of jogging women and men. Most of these little cabinettes are also provided with shade and shelter by more large, healthy trees. In fact, I loved it so much, especially feeling so snug yet so exposed at the same time that I decided to get a sleeping bag. I needed one anyway so I might as well pick up one of the best.

I knew I was going to rely on it for a long while yet and the voices agreed.

Tomorrow was payday and I went to sleep under mild skies watching the nearby naval dockyard, hoping for a brightly lit boat to drift in. Every now and then one would arrive but never when I wanted it too.

*

My personal choice for camping gear in Sydney city is Mitchell King. They have everything you need at prices even the travelling homeless can afford. I don't know why I like this store so much but I would sometimes have a look at their Army gear when I was in the Australian Army Cadets at school. Even then I was impressed with their quality, including prices and on this bright winter morning in 1994 I decided to buy one of their ex-US Army sleeping bags. Only $50.00. I also bought a US Air Force Kit Bag – $20.00 which never busted after five years of consistent use.

I bought this particular brand because I remember my father often saying, when I was small, that the US Army were far too concerned with protecting themselves and with their own comfort to be truly effective.

I think History is proving him to be basically correct.

Anyway.

The sleeping bag proved to be one of the wisest investments that I have ever made. It was very, very warm (filled with goose down) and I slept through one of Sydney's coldest winter nights in the open elements somewhere without being discomforted in the slightest.

But, like I said, it was late winter at the time, 1994 and living in the Domain, although very pleasant, was actually a health hazard – it's a good way to catch pneumonia. Another motivating factor was to not have to write with a notepad on my raised lap.

My writing was my constant companion at this time and although it was very experimental it also provided a vent for the voices who were now becoming nastier. They had already by this time claimed to have discovered God (i.e. me). This I denied at first but it explained why the voices spent their time in revealing secret philosophy to me alone. Now though, they were expecting their God to solve all of the world's problems, getting snarky when I pointed out that I couldn't even look after myself.

These voices continue to reveal secrets to me but they usually operate by providing me with questions that I have to answer. To be honest I haven't considered what will happen if I don't continue to solve these riddles. I know though, that I will lose a special power.

I cannot show you all that they have given me because there is simply not enough space for that, at the moment (and besides, it is supposed to remain secret). But I can provide a clue: if you want to cheat on any rule, be sure to cheat only some of the time. This is because in order to have or do anything, you must have the whole of that object for it to be truly effective.

But I digress.

I left the domain after two weeks and headed into Newtown looking for a squat, hoping that the Gods would smile upon me. Another advantage to a squat is that one also has company, as well as protection from nature's harshness.

When I arrived in Newtown I had absolutely no idea about how to go about finding a squat (they are advertised but in underground shops).

'JUST LOOK,' said a voice, which seemed sensible enough.

So, again, I headed away from relative safety, inveigling myself in the back alleys, sniffing the urban air for musty scents and looking for tell-tale signs of abandonment.

As it turned out, back alleys are not a good place to look for abandoned houses. You do find them, with persistence but they're usually placed right alongside the homes of the regular citizenry.

I saw no-one on this one hour hunt and when I turned onto a quiet street near Stanmore Road in Enmore I was about to give up. But then I noticed someone across the road, a long-haired teenage boy, and for some reason I realised that he was here as a guide for me, towards my present goal. There was no reason to think this but after he looked over his shoulder at me I decided to follow him, just to see. What did I have to lose?

Within five minutes I came across a clearly abandoned, large house, on Liberty Street. It looked like cosy protection from the coming cold.

My guide looked over at me when I stopped at this treasure, flabbergasted for a second time and he continued on his way.

A whole house. To myself.

Hesitantly I opened the gate expecting it to be rusted shut. It opened.

But the front door was locked and I didn't want to attract attention by smashing a window – I planned this place to be a home.

Going around the back I was overjoyed to see the kitchen door open invitingly.

Success! And Home at last!

I entered inside, expecting great things.

Chapter Five

~

Likewise Discovering Liberty

The house looked a shambles from the inside. There were large planks of wood laid haphazardly across the floor, precariously stacked up against the wall, there were shards of glass everywhere, a used butterfly needle and most of the floor boards appeared to be missing from the front hall.

But this would have to be home.

I explored deeper.

The kitchen was to the right, small and full of dishes, cups, cutlery, pots and pans, etc. They were clean though, with only a collection of dust on them.

And the tap was working. Having water on you at all times is another survival tactic for the streets, especially in this hot climate. This is because, for the squatter, it's usually safer to get out of the house during the day and only use the squat for sleeping. This lessens your chance of being caught for trespass. And being thus exposed to the hot sun and weather, without anywhere else to go, one soon learns to always have water handy. Washing was not a priority at this time.

The living room was entered through the kitchen and was already set up with a lounge set. Cleaner still than the kitchen but with its own assortment of dusty layers. The lights didn't work in here either but my supply of candles was well stocked.

After checking out the rest of the house there were: six bedrooms, three living rooms, an indoor and outdoor kitchen and two bathrooms. The bedrooms were all barren save for various colourful graffiti declaring the owners' summation of Life:

What goes around comes around!
In Karma We Trust
Occupation: Traveller, travelling with monkeys

All in all though, the house was clean and looked to be still soundly constructed – from sandstone, I think. The voices were likewise impressed and had been happily chattering away about parties, jewellery, and maybe the discovery of some cash while I was roaming over this grand castle.

I moved one of the armchairs into an adjacent bedroom to catch the sun better and opened the room's balcony doors.

What a brilliant day!

And taking out my new Bernard Malamud book, I sat in the sun, plugged in the earphones from the Walkman that I always carried on my person (the radio mixes well with the voices in my head) and began reading. I was subliminally at peace but at the same time wished I could do some writing. I had been writing so much lately, as it was my only company, that I felt drained, deep down in my core.

But reading was almost like writing, as the reader constructs their interpretation word by written word as the writer builds similarly. And for now, it was like beginning to discover a new set of friends.

*

I was awoken later that night from the beginning of sleep by a bright shining light. I sat up upon seeing it, almost instinctively, like travelling towards the blissful light that some people have witnessed having come back from Death.

But the light had a familiar odour and, raising my arm as a shield from the glare, I was quickly realising that the light probably belonged to a patrolling security guard.

'Who are you?' I asked of it.

Silence.

'You can't stay here, mate,' eventually responded a foreign accent.

I stood up and he adjusted the flash lamp so that I could see him. He was an islander, who looked somehow frightened.

'What about just for tonight,' which seemed reasonable to me.

'This is private property,' he returned, fidgeting a bit, 'you'll have to go, sorry.'

I took a step closer, to reason with him but he immediately took up a defensive stance, raising the butt of his torch.

'It's okay, mate, it's okay,' I soothed, 'I'm going. Just let me pack my bag.'

He let me do so and escorted me from the premises.

Before releasing me though, he gave me a few cigarettes and said,

'I don't like having to kick you out, son, but that's my job, you understand.'

I simply nodded, agreeing with him, essentially: it's a dirty job, but someone's gotta do it.

'I wouldn't normally do this sort of work but I've got a new family to support – that's my wife and boy in the car,' he pointed them out across the road and she waved back to him in reply.

'Don't worry; I'll find somewhere else.'

He gave me another cigarette and then left with his wife and baby son.

I looked at the house, shivering, seeing nothing preventing me from re-entering. But the guard would be back probably and he had already warned me that if he found me there again that he would call the Police.

For being feckin' HOMELESS, for Christ's sake! Sure, I was willingly such but the voices had also forced me into it by slowly sapping my entire motivation to the extent that I was not physically capable of continuing my drifting through inner city Sydney share-houses. And, like my psychiatrist later said, the desire to be homeless is in itself a symptom of schizophrenia.

Anyway.

There was a park close-by which declared, among other proclamations: 'No Camping.'

No Justice.

So I set up camp and on the verge of sleep was disturbed by about three police officers who came running through the park. When the lead officer saw me he stopped and asked if I had seen anyone running by a few moments ago.

I replied in the negative.

'You know you can't camp here, mate. We'll come back for you when we catch this fella.' And they trotted off, exercising their self-righteousness.

I went back to sleep, vaguely scared that the police would be back to haul me away. But they didn't turn up, allowing me another chance at a squat.

But what about beautiful Liberty. Should I risk returning?

Chapter Six

~

Never Doubting

Whichever squat I ended up in, I realised upon awakening, I would be running the gauntlet. So, better the devil you know.

I returned to Liberty, nervous all over and almost tangibly imagining the cops creeping up on me. But the house welcomed me back with its contemplative mildness and I soon recognised that I was safe.

In the short term.

I returned to my room (upstairs and right at the rear) and re-established my décor: lots of books, CDs in a portable rack, black Sony Discman, Walkman and various notebooks and MSS. The candles were there already but still no mattress. The cushions from the downstairs' lounge weren't comfortable either as they kept sliding out from under one during sleep.

Thus, I was back home, with Malamud.

But the voices wouldn't let me read on a chair in my room and I kept raising my head sometimes, laughing at some subconscious joke that they had loosed. Soon, they had my entire attention and to this day, 2009, I still possess them, constantly entertaining me with synchronicity.

This was basically how I spent the next six months at Liberty, out of the chill, being kicked out three times by the police but never doubting that I could return. When the voices ran out of steam I would get out a notebook and work on the problem of i: the square root of -1, which is thought to be impossible.

I began solving this problem by drawing the number plane, with 0 in the centre. I soon realised that there could be -0 and +0: the first is a consistent lack of nothing and the latter is a consistent gain of nothing, both of which are logically separate and distinct entities.

So! This simple number plane is giving up its secrets! It easily seemed to me, in my dubiously heightened state, that this new revelation was a clue, that i was not cast in blackest bedrock, like similarly to the foundation of 0.

Anyway.

I have finally worked out this solution and am currently in the process of submitting it to various science journals (Appendix A).

Don't hold your breath.

But, completely unexpectedly, some other squatters turned up with the growing warm weather of '94-95, crawling in under the high front fence. I first noticed them, sitting in the downstairs' balcony bedroom. I saw coloured blobs squeezing in through the gap in the fence. This was followed, slowly, by what could only be a safe.

The natural questions arose. Was I being invaded by other squatters? Or was this some sort of new banking project for the homeless? When the actual people started appearing I realised it was not the latter – bankers wouldn't be arguing over the safe.

After continued rising tempers, the smallest of the group, a young woman in a witch's hat, disengaged herself from the group and approached the house.

I let her in, wondering vaguely if the piercings in her lower lip hurt all that much. They made her look perpetually pouting, like the rest of the insecure.

'Hi,' I said.

'Hi. Are you squatting here?' she asked, taking off her hat and looking around the house.

'Yep.'

'Cool. Do you mind if we crash here for a while? We'll be gone in a few weeks.'

I got the distinct impression that this statement was a simple formula which nevertheless required a reassuring response if I was to avoid a vicious fight over territory. Which I would lose, being outnumbered.

'Sure, not a problem. I was getting a bit lonesome here anyway.'

'Great! What's your name?' she asked, laughing in a sombre, almost bitter manner.

'Denis.'

'I'm Galia. I'll just go and get the rest of the crew.'

Soon, she returned to her friends and managed to shut them up. They gathered up their belongings and entered their new home. We all shook hands and I decided to head up to my room in order to let them settle in. Later they brought the safe in, from what I could hear, but I don't know what happened to it finally.

There was company now and while I was walking up the stairs I had to constantly remind myself, mind your manners, mind your manners. I could not afford to not fit in with this group. If I end up ostracized at home, because of my spending time with the voices, then I'd be soon ostracized out on the bare sidewalks of Sydney.

So I let their voices mingle with mine and gradually began to look on the bright side of sharing my secure, grand mansion with complete strangers. After all, we're in the same boat together and we may as well do the work required to get along. And Galia looked like someone who could appreciate my stories, or at least tell me what needed improvement.

I fell asleep to the sound of music and a roaring fire.

Chapter Seven

~

The Anti-Psychotics Help

Expecting breakfast the following morn, I headed downstairs and followed the sound of music emanating from the front hallway bedroom.

'Morning,' I greeted the young couple.

'Hi,' returned the female. 'Do you like punk?'

'It's still pure genius,' I replied.

She harrumphed and looked back down at the book she was reading. Her boyfriend was laying in her lap, very happy in his quiet contemplation.

Breakfast would have to be garnered somehow. Food was the biggest bill for me, on Sydney's streets, mainly because I had no cooking facilities and wasn't living close to any free food, as in Melbourne. I could only have takeaway or restaurant service. There was also tobacco and alcohol but never enough for as much as you wanted.

So I chose to beg, or 'scam' as I called it, in order to eat.

I still do not know if begging is ethically acceptable to me but I am now redeeming my doubt by regularly giving to buskers and charity.

Of course this begging was also a deep lesson in human behaviour since most of the people that I approached for 'a dollar' were simply too self-centred to be generous. And I still ask when any new unexpected event arises, why does most of humanity invariably seek the most negative path?

I don't know.

Anyway, I got that morning's breakfast kebab and the rest of the pleasant day was waiting to be planned. I could continue with the maths, maybe muck around with some prose, or scam up some more money for beers.

I decided to just return home and wait for the rest of the house to return.

I really was lonely.

*

The couple with the stereo, Erica and Jamieson, who still wears his very untidy Mohawk, didn't really feel like talking. So I entered the living room and sat down with my hypotheses about Collapsibility Theory, which basically complements Calculus.

Anyway.

I began to draw another, different, number plane and then noticed a large advertisement placed on the mantelpiece, upon seeking a new centre for this mathematical creation:

BAD JOKES: 20c
VERY BAD JOKES: 25c

When they returned home I asked about the sign.

'That's mine,' said Stephen (I later learned his name and the rest of theirs).

'Do you want to buy a joke?'

'Can I get one on credit?'

He thought about that, looking up and off to his left and then soon replied.

'Sure. What do you call someone with a seagull on their head?'

'What?'

'Cliff!'

I personally thought that this was very funny, and I soon gave him the 20c for the joke. He made a bit of money that way, if the rumours are true, with another such sign out with him on the streets. At least enough to get by.

*

At an impromptu house meeting called by Galia one night soon after they took up residency, in order to fix up the house, she volunteered to do the cooking, if the boys (three) took care of the basic renovation. We asked her to tie back her ancient green dreads if she expected us to accept her labours. She was pleased by the compliment, as we all surmised and then asked us when could we begin?

We seriously pondered this unexpected nutter and eventually Stephen applied Occam's razor:

'We've got a fire and a pot. We can just boil the meat and the pasta or whatever and be well able to survive. We'd live like Kings.'

'And Queens,' rightly pointed out Sonya. Sonya was one of the rare homeless people who also had a job. Exactly what doing, I no longer remember but she apparently travelled around Australia, working and living in squats. She was also perpetually to be seen with a bottle of expensive wine whenever she was at home.

We naturally also developed a loose set of rules which we all, bar one (who shall remain nameless), adhered to reasonably well. I was the only one who remained at home during the day, while the rest got out into the heart of the city.

The promised bounty though we could not fully manage, nor the rigorous renovation we had planned and everybody tended to spend their evenings around the hearth, over a cask of wine talking, playing with the fire and mucking around with the stereo.

We followed pretty much the same pattern for the next two years, being regularly evicted every three months or so. At one stage Galia, her visitors and I even took to living in the roof, which was accessible from an outside attic door, across the back patio roof from the outside kitchen without its railings.

Galia and I still remain in contact to this day, having accidentally met in Newtown a couple of years ago now. She's going great guns with her own fashion label which sells reasonably well at festivals all around the country. One shop has even recently asked her for more of her T-shirts to sell.

But what especially endeared her to me was the small way she had of looking after me, even though both of us were in the worst of civilised worlds. Basically, soon after she moved in, she would leave two cigarettes for me to wake up to on her way out into the city. I think, really, only smokers can appreciate this gesture, as I sometimes did not have the means with which to satisfy my cravings upon waking. Thus, feeling normal again, I could head out for breakfast and to decide which book to read for the day. When I returned I would have enough tobacco and enough money – all thanks to Galia's initial forethought. Incredible!

The police had their desired effect though, I found myself alone in Liberty again and living under the floor – it was the last place they thought of looking and they only sometimes gave it a cursory inspection through the knee high opening at the side of the house.

Throughout these three years of residence at Liberty, ending in about the summer of 1997, I was also in and out of various psychiatric hospitals, usually to steer clear of the cops after another raid. I would be in there for about six weeks at a time, slowly getting these crazy voices under control but I never followed up with the medication after discharge. I simply didn't think that I was mentally ill: I still believe this but the anti-psychotics now help to handle my eccentricities and the voices.

Anyway, I finally left Liberty behind when I was awoken by the sound of roaring fire. It sounded exactly like running water and I wasn't sure which was which until I heard a siren approaching. I quickly evacuated, leaving everything behind, to be met by a police officer being guided to my hidey-hole by a neighbour.

She escorted me out to the front footpath and explained that the indoor stairs had been set alight. I hadn't heard nor seen anything, I told her and wasn't sure if I was even awake and hearing running water/fire.

She let me go and told me that I would have to find new 'accommodation' (I think she actually used that word). Almost tearfully, I re-packed my bag with its full assortment of belongings and headed off to the heart of Newtown looking for another home.

Liberty left behind, to learn the King Street Blues.

Chapter Eight

~

To Mingle with Passers-By

Heading down King Street, Newtown, sweating and worried, hoping one of its cross streets held a safe squat, I remembered something Stephen said before leaving Liberty (he was the first to go).

'There's a powered squat at __ Newman Street. I'm gonna try there.'

Considering that I had spent some time at Newman Boys' High School, it seemed obvious that the elements were calling me to a new home.

But where is Newman Street?

I asked at a real estate agent and was soon approaching a ramshackle house with its front door clearly hanging off its hinges. There was also the sound of a transistor radio issuing from the front room.

I approached cautiously.

So far, so good. Now just up the front steps.

Almost falling through the second one, to peek my head around the front entrance.

There was a straw blonde, long haired man inside. He appeared to be wrapped solely in a thin blanket. There was also a respectable fire blazing in the hearth, despite the heat of the day.

'G'day!'

He looked up and smiled, continuing his secretly encoded arm and fingers discussion.

'Can I crash here? My squat burned down.'

He nodded and guided me through the rest of the house with a sweeping gesture of his left, vibrant arm.

The house was small, made from wooden planks with largish gaps between them. The living room was piled high throughout with all manner of male and female clothing. It was all clean too. Part of the space was taken up by a futon mattress which I claimed as mine. I rummaged through the clothing and duly discovered the warm blankets that were hidden there.

There was one other bedroom, a kitchen, a bathroom and a garage. The second bedroom also contained a mattress and it was difficult to tell if its assorted bric-a-brac belonged to a current, or past resident.

And so, after unpacking my kitbag, I decided to introduce myself more properly to my neighbour.

I wasn't expecting just any 'normal' conversation but to discover another new perspective, with expressions and concepts similar to my own voices and to appreciate the Universe more fundamentally: for madness has indeed a method.

'Hi,' I said, after knocking on his doorpost.

He looked up and smiled.

'My name is Denis. Mind if I join you for a while?'

He ushered me closer.

I took out my tobacco and offered him some. He refused.

So I rolled a smoke and began on familiar ground: the weather. He preferred the cooler weather, because of its Gods and Goddesses. I can no longer remember his exact words, even vaguely, for they bespoke of vast Empires and Gods beyond this ken of mine. He was, though, proud and clear about the fact that he was a painter, his paints and brushes being still packed away, he said.

He subsequently, around one week later, impressed his artisanship upon me by painting a perfect rendition of a Phoenix arising from the ashes. It covered the entire length of the wall containing his 'door'. Its bright green and long elegant wingspan with firmly detailed feathers also reminded the viewer of dry desert mysteries, speaking in new, legible hieroglyphics. I don't know where he could have possibly obtained that much paint and there certainly was not enough empty paint cans (which were all small, 100g containers) to fully justify the job.

Well, like I said earlier, there's a method, there's a method, somewhere, there is always a method.

Trent, however, was sad, and fidgeted with each of my compliments. Finally, I asked him if he thought it was as good as I did.

It was, he said but it contained one fatal flaw: it wasn't portable, or was that sort of the point?

Neither of us knew, so I left him to his unhappy perspective and unable to tell him myself that every 'bad' event can be viewed as an opportunity. But, still, that thought has to be worked at, constantly reminding oneself that he/she is growing positively and not paying heed to that negative little voice.

I, however, returned to the kitchen and immediately began revelling in the simple boiling of water in a kettle and the subsequent pouring of coffee. I plugged in the speakers to my Discman, turned it on and invited the voices to a party.

The voices love a party, no matter how grumpy that they might be at the time of invitation and when they start mingling with passers'-by voices then Reality reveals a more positive aspect.

And, again, this is how I spent the next six months at Newman Street: talking with the voices alone at home. Some days though the voices would wake up nasty, which would soon require admission to the nearest psychiatric hospital.

These things do tend to pile up without maintenance.

Anyway.

Chapter Nine

~

And Another Roaring Fire

For the third time now I awoke to the sound of a roaring fire. Am I meant to take this as some sort of hint?

It was late morning, mild and clear, spring '98.

I could have raised myself but I chose to assume that Trent was in complete charge of festivities. I was assured that he was indeed calmly present by the sound of his quiet conversation with someone. Was it the owner of the second bedroom? There was also the sound of snapping wood, presumably feeding the fun.

The oncoming sirens, followed by a very throaty engine, soon raised other possibilities. Still, I would not get up. Everybody else could solve this one.

Which they did, to their credit and as quietly as possible. It was when the cops arrived that the dramas began. I didn't know that they had turned up but when Trent yelled out that the DSS had cut him off long ago, taking his only I.D., I pretended to be asleep, in humble protest and resistance at this ungentlemanly inspection.

'Is there anyone else in the house?' loudly questioned the deep voice of bigotry, properly dressed and pressed, I'm sure.

'I can't remember,' Trent replied.

The cops thumped their way forwards.

'Hey fella! Wake up!'

I let him stew.

He kicked the bottom of the mattress.

I turned over, calling out my one true love's name.

That shut him up for a while.

'Fella, if you don't wake up I'm going to have to kick you all out.'

He was going to kick us out nevertheless, to justly protect all private property, which is the central tenet of any cop's job.

So I remained asleep, wondering if he would pick up the hint that this was the only place that I had to sleep in.

'Right...'

'Wha...?' I said, suddenly bolting upright. I still had my eyes closed.

'Mate, I've gotta see your I.D.'

I opened my eyes while turning to my wallet by the left of the large bed.

I showed him my DSS I.D., which he duly noted. Handing it back he said,

'You can't stay here, fella. This is private property. Have you got somewhere else to go to?'

'No.'

'Well, you'll find somewhere. I'm sure you always do.'

I smiled in response: real helpful, wasn't he?

Anyway, he guided me outside to the footpath to join Trent and the second, nameless resident, who always came home late and left early, with a heavy sports bag. At least we had collected some of the warm clothing from the floor of the squat.

We didn't say much and I was the first to leave the group. None of us particularly felt like going back because we had all been individually and officially warned against renewing our trespass. This was unusual since most of the time the cops never bothered to check up on our continued squatting.

It's a very rare squat that has electricity, mattresses, blankets and clothing if you want it. I was mulling this over while headed in a predestined direction.

Another abandoned house near Newman Street.

Upon a previous cursory test of its various entrances, this brick house appeared to be locked up solid. But I had noticed some planks missing from the side fence revealing a large, wild garden. This time I stepped in deeper.

No-one would see me sleeping in that tall grass.

Perfect!

I set up base at the back of the garden but soon realised that I would need some sort of sleeping mat.

So I headed into Newtown and picked up a few boxes of waxed cardboard. I went back for a few extra when I noticed a few drops from a sudden storm.

This was going to be novel – safely snug in the heart of the thrashing wild.

But I did not settle easily into this campsite, feeling very exposed, with only the nervous US Army and cardboard for defence.

What made it worse was having to look at the boarded up entrance at the back of the house.

'So close and yet so far.'

But the voices soon suggested a way to protect myself in this very hostile environment. Light a candle and throw it over the fence while yelling,

'DYNAMITE!'

It was basically the only idea in town at that stage and I relied on the fact that a lit candle bears somewhat of a resemblance to dynamite. Besides, having such vulnerable 'housing' necessitated some pro-active defence.

So I flung the 'dynamite' over the fence:

'DYNAMITE!'

Appropriately, some scuffling footsteps duly quickened.

It's all in the mind.

But now, I had to worry about the SWAT team turning up. I was already hearing nagging, persistent voices and radio crackle claiming to be detectives investigating God so the combination of the two led to a sleepless, terrorized night under a vigorous storm, flicking me with water and debris. The cardboard basically worked though.

Eventually I closed my eyes and managed somehow to tune out from the voices, longing for dawn in a quiet, calm semi-doze.

I wished I could get into that house.

Chapter Ten

~

Clearly Visible

There was a surprise waiting for me after I had finished my morning cigarette and donned my glasses – the corrugated iron sheet had been completely removed from the backyard entrance to the house. There remained only another sheet blocking off the lower half of the opening, easily climbed over.

Accordingly, I thanked the Gods and eagerly repacked my small baggage. I left the cardboard where it was.

But at the point of entry I had the overwhelming conviction that this could be a trap set by the cops to catch the begging homeless. I had no proof of such, yet still cautiously began my desired exploration.

It was not a trap, just a thoroughly abandoned house covered in heavy layers of grey dust, missing most of the flooring and walls from the upstairs bedrooms. The inside of the roof gables were also clearly visible, with their nooks inhabited by cooing pigeons.

Again, I established myself in what appeared to be the living room, containing the revealed opening.

I had also, several days ago, noticed a double-bed mattress, apparently pristine, discarded outside a clothing bin nearer the first Newman Squat than this present one and now decided to take ownership of it.

It was while taking the short walk for this treasure that my lifestyle began to appear in its true light: completely hopeless and barely hanging together, like my house. In fact the more I thought about it, the more desperate appeared my plight.

This was an emergency. Necessitating direct action. Non-violent, and psychic of course.

Thus, I took up the semi-lotus position upon the centre of my new and only piece of furniture. I looked directly at the trickling pedestrians with all of my predicament and struggle registered upon my facial features. Most of them smiled in response but how could they really help?

In due course two police officers on pushbikes turned up which was the expected proof that my psychic protest at the lack of reasonable housing had been indeed registered with the relevant authorities. The lead officer looked me over sitting there peacefully channelling my newly discovered outrage. He looked away and they both cycled down the facing perpendicular street.

I felt great: help was on its way!

I decided to reward myself with a bottle of whisky. After finally getting the mattress into the house I headed out to scam up some extra money for the festivities.

Begging money from complete strangers is a numbers game. The more people you ask the more cash you can collect. Gratefully as well, the large majority of people in Newtown did not berate me for this begging, choosing instead to simply say no. This is fair enough, in hindsight, as the world would be a very tacky place if it was full of ultra-nice guys and gals handing out lollies and lucre to all and sundry. Where would society's motivation be then?

Of course, one has to be creative with the way one approaches the common person for 'a dollar.' My personal tactic is to say that the money is for a phone card. Saying that it's 'for a feed' tends to be less successful.

These times spent begging, I recall now, were usually the only time that I came into contact with the regular citizenry. The rest of the time I spent talking with the voices, alone in my squat. Occasionally, I would be forced to break this crazy monotony with some writing or some maths but usually I was talking with the voices through the radio in my Walkman. Great fun!

Anyway, after a couple of hours I had enough money for the celebration and decided on the rare treat of buying some groceries – bread, margarine, a small tin of salmon and a can opener. This latter would have to also double as a butter knife.

The oil from the salmon stained the new mattress but I chose to view it as a psychic continuation of today's protest. The trouble was though, that I could not completely rely on the apparent proof provided by the earlier arrival of the police that my protest had been indeed heard. As with all psychic proof it was simply not reliable. Even though I had predicted it consciously making myself aware of what to expect as proof.

So the oil stain would have to act as a constant subconscious encouragement to return to the mainstream and to live the pleasant life that I was starting to become envious of. A life evident everywhere on my short excursions.

Anyway.

My woes could wait for the time being and I decided to plug the speakers into the radio in order to better get the feeling that I was at a vibrant party.

Thus I drank and danced the night away, encouraging the voices from the Walkman to distract me from these new feelings of abandonment.

Things would have to change. And quickly.

Chapter Eleven

~

As the Garden of Eden

The radio was still playing when I groggily awoke the following afternoon. I turned it off and went back to sleep.

Hunger eventually revived me in the early evening and after my last remaining cigarette I considered again the options that I had last night devised in order to get away from this desperate life.

GO BACK TO HOSPITAL, proclaimed the voices unanimously. This was a practically guaranteed path to secure accommodation, as every psychiatric hospital has a social worker to assist its homeless patients into reasonable accommodation. I had learned this first hand in my previous admissions into psych. hospitals but had always believed a squat was quite adequate for my needs. I also lacked the necessary motivation to actively pursue decent housing, which I could not admit to anybody and so took the easier path of squatting.

Despite its obvious benefits however, I was not willing to go back there and willingly suffer my freedom being abrogated by their putting me in the locked ward again, even though it was only for the first two or three weeks of my stay.

There was one man in the locked ward at Rozelle Hospital, Tom, who had been there for three years since about 1995. I naturally felt sorry for him but when he asked to see my penis one day, persistently, I figured out what his problem was.

I hope he's still locked up.

But, by the same token, I told myself while scamming up my breakfast kebab in the warm evening, I was not willing to continue living the itinerant life. This point I began to drum into my subconscious by sleeping every night with my arm laid protectively across my head, in case the roof fell in on me. After a short while this had the desired effect and I came to the conclusion, about a week later, that if I continued to stay in this unstable house my life would continue to be threatened. Physically.

'YOU WILL EASILY DIE UNDER A SHARP PILE OF RUBBLE.'

I duly evacuated and admitted myself to Rozelle Hospital. The Missenden Unit (the psychiatric wing of RPAH) was closer but I've always preferred the large, leafy grounds at Rozelle. I used to think of it as the Garden of Eden.

Anyway, this turned out to be my first shaky step towards relative stability.

*

My voices had also become very vicious by then, instructing me to commit suicide, because I had been dealing in ancient magick (i.e. basically solving every problem that the voices asked of me). I believed these voices and their questioning nature and on my walk to the hospital did my best to fulfil their wishes.

I gave up after I lay my head on the centre of the road, looking away from oncoming traffic, hoping someone would be kind enough to put me out of my mental misery.

A car was approaching.

It slowed down and then stopped. The passenger door creaked open, like a grave and I heard the crackle of the police radio.

Footsteps approached.

'Are you okay, mate?'

I did not reply. Just run me over.

'Have you lost something?'

'My mind.'

'Pardon?'

I sat up, hearing only his lack of concern.

I looked up at him.

'Sorry, officer but I thought if no one killed me soon then I'd head into hospital to find help.'

'Would you like us to take you there?'

'I'd prefer to do it myself.'

'Well see that you do.' And the wagon drove off.

I considered remaining where I was, to hope for some motor driven guillotine but the arrival of the cops I took as a sign that my death was not yet warranted. It was a slim hope and only sufficed to get me admitted into the hospital.

Surprisingly though, they didn't put me in the locked ward, even though I was clearly a danger to myself. I was admitted into Ward 25, an open ward. I spent a sleepless night there, grateful for the shelter but trying to commit suicide with my imagination. When that didn't work I pulled out all bar three of my dreadlocks which somehow calmed me down enough (maybe it was the shock of the pain) to wait for breakfast peacefully.

How I longed for the beautiful light of dawn.

*

The voices got their wish after breakfast, in the bright chilliness.

I threw myself in front of an oncoming milk truck. When the ambulance arrived they discovered a collapsed right lung and rushed me to RPAH.

I was soon seen by a medical team, the doctor of which told me that they would have to insert a tube down my throat in order to re-inflate my lung.

I concurred expecting the worst.

I duly gagged on the tube and they were forced to cut a small whole in the side of my chest if I was to continue breathing.

And success, finally!

*

I spent a few weeks recuperating and was eventually admitted to the Missenden Unit under the Mental Health Act.

I had learned my lesson. By hook or by crook I am staying off of the killer streets.

Chapter Twelve

~

Belonging to Me

Gradually and with Luck's help, a simple plan emerged. Of course, I could have just pursued the social worker but my previous experiences with them had not been enthusing.

What I did decide upon however was to find a fellow patient at Missenden, who could somehow put me into safe housing.

The most likely patient presented himself: Jeffrey Applegate. We met casually enough over morning coffee at 6am (after I had been discharged to the open ward) and he told me that he had a two bedroom flat.

'Who's staying in the second bedroom?' I asked.

'No one.'

Brilliant!

'Do you mind if I stay there?'

'That'd be great; it gets pretty lonely there all by myself.'

And so it was settled. I informed my hospital psychiatrist that I had found somewhere to stay but when he learned the details he informed me that the hospital did not encourage patients to move in with each other, as this usually led to disaster of one sort or another.

So I capitulated, telling my psychiatrist that I'd ask the social worker to find me a place somewhere.

A few weeks later, just before my discharge, the social worker (I have no idea of her name) told me that the best she could come up with, for someone without bond, was Hope Hostel, Westmead. They charged $12.50 per night.

'Do you have enough to get you by there until payday?' she asked.

'Yes.' The truth was I had no money, as Jeffrey had borrowed most of it, apparently to get some of his things out of the pawn shop. He paid half of it back over the course of our stay at Missenden.

I'm still waiting for the rest.

Nevertheless I was discharged a couple of days later, presumably to Hope Hostel, when in fact Jeffrey had already given me the keys to take up residency at his place.

And thus I set off to Marrickville to partake of an easier life.

*

I had no trouble finding the flat and after unpacking my bag I felt completely out of water. Thinking that this immaculately clean flat, with its well-stocked refrigerator, belonged to me now as well was somewhat of a culture shock.

Nor did I really get over it. Most of the time in this new place I spent sleeping (having exhausted my maths and writing) only rising for breakfast and dinner.

Jeffrey also told me to have replaced the groceries that I used by the time he got back. This seemed fair enough and I began, after a few days home, by replacing the Weet-Bix and fruit that I had partaken of. I would get around to the meat and bread, etc. later on.

This of course never happened and I spent about a week and a half living on cereal and fruit, once a day. The rest of the time I slept, or tried to concentrate on some television.

Jeffrey arrived home and I synchronistically opened the front door for him. What made this the more remarkable was the fact that I was not usually up and about at that time of day.

He threw his bag onto the sofa and went straight for the fridge. He also checked the freezer which, luckily, I was too unmotivated to even suspect that it existed.

'Why didn't you leave the meat out?' he wailed.

'Oh, I'm sorry, I forgot,' I thought.

I can read minds so, of course, I should have known he would come home when he did. Silly me!

'I didn't look in the freezer,' I replied.

And things went downhill from there.

After dinner (which Jeffrey prepared) he asked me to somehow get $20 to replace the groceries.

'I'll ring up my father tomorrow,' I agreed.

'You have to get it now.' It was either that or get thrown out on the streets again.

I rang up my father.

He was extremely glad to hear from me, not knowing where I was after being told that I was going to Hope Hostel.

I asked him for the money and added,

'Maybe I should go to Rozelle?'

Rozelle Psychiatric Hospital had always saved my bacon before, so now they can bloody well find me a place, instead of continually discharging me back to unstable housing.

Dad soon turned up and we quickly got my things together for the return to safety. As were leaving Jeffrey came running out, yelling,

'Excuse me, Mr. Fitzpatrick?'

Dad stopped, and turned around.

'Yes,' he replied.

'Would you have twenty bucks to replace the food that Denis ate while he was here?' Jeffrey looked in the throes of a secret addiction.

'Sure,' Dad asserted, 'no problem.'

He revealed his inner coat pocket and produced a wad of fifties. Mum quickly made him put it away and said to the obviously agitated Jeffrey,

'I'm sorry, we can't help you.' Which Jeffrey couldn't gainsay.

We left instantly, with Jeffrey staring at us open mouthed and we were soon off to the Garden of Eden.

This was my final, surer, step towards a place belonging to me exclusively.

Chapter Thirteen

~

Rapt and Speechless

As with any admission we had to wait for about half an hour before seeing the admitting psychiatrist. We spent the intervening time with my father outlining how I should never have been previously discharged back to my various squats, legally. This was a constant theme of his on the rare, former occasions that we had talked but this time I was willing to listen. And the more I listened the more I felt a subconscious sense of growing outrage.

But still, I reminded myself, I had been on a quest, discovering as a result latent psychic abilities which everyone innately possesses.

This of course could not be believed, out of hand, by most psychiatrists, even when you point out to them that a flock of birds changes direction with one mind, as does a school of fish.

Anyway.

The doctor, somewhat rotund and jolly looking, made an appearance finally and guided us to her office.

My father did most of the talking, concentrating on my past discharges and how this was not conducive to my mental health which the doctor quickly agreed to. She suggested placing me in Rehabilitation (to teach one living skills again, like cooking, cleaning, budgeting, etc.) after about six weeks in an open ward. And if I coped well in Rehab., then the hospital would get me into affordable accommodation.

I was rapt and speechless and simply nodded when the psychiatrist asked me if I would agree to this plan.

Thus, I was soon transferred to ward 26, which was my centre in Eden, having stayed there contentedly on my previous admissions into Rozelle. My parents left when they saw that I was secured, giving me twenty dollars for the drink machine, etc.

I went to bed soon after, imagining a little apartment in the future.

*

I spent about six weeks in ward 26 and, like every other admission, my residency there was one sustained party. I went AWOL repeatedly to buy beers but was always sure to report back to the head nurse and only drink with a few select patients, deep in the hospital grounds. I also bought several packets of breath mints to cover up the alcohol on our breath but our little group didn't really need much alcohol anyway to get us inebriated – we mentally ill are very sensitive.

I was officially registered as a voluntary patient about three weeks after admission which meant that I could go and come as I pleased, only needing to inform a nurse upon egress and arrival. It also meant that the nurses didn't have to fill out the copious AWOL forms that they were constantly nagging me about.

*

After about six weeks in ward 26 my treating psychiatrist told me that I would be going into Rehab. within the next few days.

'And if I go well in there will you find me a place?'

'That's still the plan,' she replied.

I was transferred two days later, in the afternoon, in time for dinner.

Even the food was better there and more of it. What wonders would there be for breakfast?

I spent my first night there watching television and meeting my fellow neighbours.

THIS PLACE TRULY IS PARADISE. I had to agree with the voices there.

I went to bed at about 10pm and slept the sleep of the innocent.

Chapter Fourteen

~

To This Day

As with Jeffrey's place I found it hard to accept that anybody could significantly help me here in Rehab. Not only with a decent dwelling but with the persistent voices who were angry at me for not dying as a result of my stunt with the milk truck. Consequently I spent most of my time there sleeping, interacting rarely with the staff and patients but eating well nonetheless.

And slowly, through sheer bastard mettle, I realised that I only had myself to rely on, that I was the only one capable of helping myself. I was fed up with only being able to sleep and considered again a secret wish of mine – to sell my books from door to door. It was a goal I gained as the result of being a travelling sales rep. with Macmillan Publishing.

This could give me something to live for. The more I thought about it the more hyped-up I became. I didn't have to produce books just yet though but I could sell one page stories for a dollar each. In fact it might be the beginning of a new genre.

And this was how I began my successful self-publishing career. I was actually forced into it one hot day in 1998 when I ran out of tobacco and had to wait a few days for payday. Having no money at all brought my goal into a new perspective.

In light of which I quickly wrote up ten thoroughly experimental pieces, handwritten, folded into an A5 booklet with a surreal Celtic knot work border on each page. The choice of the text being handwritten was very deliberate. It was written in such a way that different people would interpret the handwriting differently, creating a plethora of stories from the one source.

I took these 10 stories into Leichhardt and sold 6 of them for $2 each. $12. Enough to get a small pouch lasting three days.

I headed for the supermarket realising in subliminal glee that I could make money from my writing.

I bought the tobacco, even getting back some change.

For the next three days that pouch was a constant reminder that I could live off of my creations and I soon threw myself into the task of writing some traditional fiction, or at least writing that could be more easily comprehended. I stayed up longer, building up a collection of stories to sell in Newtown. I also decided to participate in some of the organised activities and found a few people to provide criticism on my work.

I didn't realise I was improving, nor that the voices were becoming tamer again.

*

After about six months in Rehab. I was transferred into one of the five cottages on the grounds. This was the official last step before I could be discharged back into the community.

Unlike before I had no trouble recognising that this cottage was my own to look after, a fact emphasized by my requirement to pay market rent on the place. 'Fair enough,' I thought, 'I'll have to pay rent wherever I go.'

I spent my time there mostly sleeping which is a defence of mine to change, or prolonged stress.

When I got over this initial period of adjustment I started self-publishing again. This time it was booklets of poetry but written with a computer. I didn't sell much, just enough to buy me a pouch of tobacco whenever I ran out of options to refresh my addiction.

Buying the right amount of food to last the entire fortnight was a bit of a trick for me to master. Nor did I get the hang of it during my entire stay there, to the point where one of my flat mates, Trevor, would criticize me for not buying food at the weekly house meetings. It wasn't like I was eating their food, I just don't eat much. The other three flatmates had no problem with me but we all tended to live in our own little worlds and engaged each other from that perspective.

There was one memorable day however, during the chill of '99, when the voices encouraged me to go into Newtown to celebrate ANZAC day. Their take on the matter was that I too had been involved in a war, a psychological war, to discover fundamental meaning within myself and within the Universe. This had been proven with the discovery of my psychic abilities which give me the sense that Life is worth living.

I got to Newtown train station at about 2pm and it seemed that almost every lamppost on King Street was hosting a game of two up. And the money people were throwing around! Wads of fifties and hundreds seemed to take life and fly about in the cold damp.

There was one man though who seemed at odds with his setting. I noticed him, walking down towards the station, looking the modern beatnik, with his left arm held up in the air while he walked. As he got closer I could see that he was holding $10 out to the quickest taker in the crowd. But the crowd assumed that he meant something else, leaving the money for me to grab as he passed by. Nothing was said at my boldness which still leaves me with the impression that he was indeed bequeathing a gift.

I continued on my way deciding to visit the Oxford Hotel with my windfall. I also had some money of my own and, with one thing leading to another, I left the Oxford at closing time stumbling my way back to hospital.

They weren't impressed at my racket upon finding I had lost my keys. But I was voluntary and after assuring them that it was my first drink in several weeks, they doubtfully forgave me. I then cut out future drinking, not willing to risk my promised land.

I was just getting used to the house when the social worker, Andrea, called on me one day, with unbelievable news.

After the initial greetings she began.

'Remember the application we put in to the Department of Housing two weeks ago?'

'Yes.' I had no faith whatsoever in that Dept., having previously applied and been put on a ten year waiting list.

'Well, they've offered you a bed-sitter.'

I grabbed the light.

'Great! When can I move in?'

'First things first. You have to inspect it to decide whether or not you agree that it's inhabitable. If you don't like it they'll offer you only one more place which you either have to take or forgo. How does that sound?'

'Just as long as the roof isn't about to collapse, I'll take the first one.' She laughed and arranged a time to have a look at the place.

Success!

*

We visited the place two days later after picking up the keys. It was very clean, compact and also contained a washing machine. The lights were working, the tap didn't drip and swivelled easily. There was no racket from loud and raucous neighbours either.

'Like I said Andrea, I'll take it.'

'Excellent! Well, congratulations, Denis, you've certainly earned it after putting up with so many obstacles.'

'It keeps me on my toes.'

And to this day I remain sheltered, having upgraded to a still better address.

I also sued Central Sydney Area Health Service, in about 2007 for their breach of duty of care in continuously discharging me back into unsafe accommodation. I won and the compensation has helped me establish my own personal Garden of Eden.

I have learned a lot.

Appendix A

~

Hypothetically Calibrated i

© Denis Fitzpatrick, BA, 1989 - 2006

Considering recent discussions regarding possible variability in fundamental constants, such as the speed of light (1), one is thereby provided with an environment of change in which to consider finding whether one can have a potentially calibrated i (i.e. i being algebraic for the square root of -1, which does not have two negative roots that easily reconcile.) i is a subliminal problem (since about the 5th Century AD, beginning in Islam) for Mathematicians and Physicists since it states that i is imaginary, in the sense that: to be later understood with a fresh understanding of $x^2 = +/-1$.

And one says again: i is hardly considered to be a problem; the answer is 'coming up.' Yet it is known that the complex systems underpinning the

Universe are sensitive to even the slightest change, and, considering recent discussions regarding the actual possible variability of the fundamental constant, alpha, the bond between electrons and protons, called the fine structure constant, considering such discussions, the promised solution to i, 'in the future', is to be naturally pondered, now, with a view to some reasonable answer. It is even possibly another effect of a variable alpha, and bound to consequently arise.

Note, naturally, the accepted, almost categorically, fundamental objection and observation (i.e. ...'the mathematical description of N3 is not F = -F') regarding the equations herein under observed between F = -F, allowing one to thereby potentially resolve i, contains no difference between the Known variable/constant and the Unknown variable/constant. Such difference is observed plainly everywhere though.

Thus, when one applies Newton's Third Law of Motion (that every action has an equal and opposite reaction) to the problem of solving, or perhaps testing, i, one further notes:

F(body A on body B) action direction = -F(body B on body A) reaction direction

1 Newton (body A on body B) action direction = -1 Newton (body B on body A) reaction direction

Therefore, (sqrt 1) Newton (body A on body B) action direction = (sqrt -1) Newton (body B on body A) reaction direction

In other words (therefore), (sqrt -1) Newton (body B on body A) reaction direction = (sqrt 1) Newton (body A on body B) action direction
= 1 Newton (body A on body B) action direction, or
-1 Newton (body B on body A) reaction direction
= 1 Newton (body A on body B) action direction, in most cases.

One can thus certainly expect a possibly new direction for Electrical Engineering, among other things, realised now, rather than postponed as being future soluble.

(1) Universe.nasa.gov/press/2003/031124a.html

About the Author

I began my publishing career with handwritten, avant-garde works. The handwritten choice was deliberate as different readers would read my scrawl differently, thus arriving at an interpretation unique to each. Surprisingly, these works sold well and I decided to take myself seriously. I was a patient in Rozelle Psychiatric Hospital at this time.

I was soon after discharged from the Hospital and bequeathed a Dept of Housing bed-sitter, after five years of homelessness (late 1998). After writing up some novice short stories and buying a second-hand electronic typewriter, I chose what I thought was the best of them, typed them out, photocopied them in batches of twenty at Newtown Public Library to be sold in Newtown for $1.00 each. A new batch every so often.

Again, these projects were very successful and my father eventually talked me into taking some stories to Snap Printing and having them professionally printed and saddle-stitched. My second self-published project (*Watching Every Colour: Selected Fitzpatrick* © Denis Fitzpatrick, 2004) was picked up by the publisher Independence Jones, who promptly offered me a verbal publishing contract for a collection of short stories (*Bearing All Gods and Goddesses*, © Denis Fitzpatrick, 2004).

Finally, a journalist from *The Sydney Morning Herald* picked up some of my efforts and consequently wrote up a very favourable review of my literary style and unique marketing technique to passers-by.

This book is the hopefully still more of the best to come.

Denis Fitzpatrick, BA
Sydney, Australia
August 2006